HIPPOCRATES
Health Program

HIPPOCRATES
Health Program

A Proven Guide to Healthful Living

DR. BRIAN R. CLEMENT

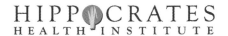

Library of Congress Cataloging-in-Publication Data

ISBN-13: 978-0-9622-3730-0 (Paperback)
ISBN-10: 0-9622-3730-2 (Paperback)

© 2014 Brian R. Clement, PhD

Publisher: Hippocrates Health Institute
      1443 Palmdale Court
      West Palm Beach, FL 33411

Cover design by Larissa Hise Henoch
Inside design and formatting by Larissa Hise Henoch

• • •

To the caring people of the Earth,
To the children, and to the magnificent creatures
who share this planet with us.

• • •

Contents

DEDICATION v

FOREWORD ix

John Robbins
> Author of *Diet For a New America* and *President of EarthSave*

INTRODUCTION xi

1. HOW OUR FOOD AFFECTS OUR LIFE 1
> A history Leadership and Innovations/
> How We Have Deviated/Why Living and Raw Food—
> The Basics of Nourishment

2. THE RE-EMERGENCE OF AN OLD TRUTH 7
> Super nutrition through Germinating and Sprouting/
> Wheatgrass—the Green Miracle/Tray Greens/
> the Value of Juices/Dehydrated and Fermented Foods

3. OPTIMUM ASSIMILATION AND DIGESTION 17
> Proper Food Combining/Eliminative
> Health/Fasting

4. EXPANDING THE PARAMETERS 21
> Sunlight, Air and Water/Detoxify Your
> Home/Clothing/Planetary Wellness

5. THE EXERCISE IMPERITIVE.................................31

6. BODY/MIND/SPIRIT—UNFOLDING
   INTO WELLNESS.......................................35

7. MODERN DILEMMAS 39
   Addictions/Hypoglycemia/Candida
   Albicans

8. WHAT TO EXPECT FROM OTHERS.....................45

9. INDIVIDUALIZING THE DIET.......................49

CONCLUSION...55

HIPPOCRATES OFFERS AN UNSURPASSED
HEALTH PROGRAM 61

HEALTH EDUCATOR CERTIFICATION 63

LIFE TRANSFORMATION PROGRAM 64

EQUIPMENT NEEDED TO IMPLEMENT THE LIVE
   FOOD PROGRAM 65

HIPPOCRATES PUBLICATIONS.......................67

FOOTNOTES...69

Foreword

Today there is a wave of "awakening" sweeping across the earth. More and more people are realizing that in deviating from the natural order, we have lost something precious' but, if we live according to the universal laws, we can recover what has been lost and attain the great blessing of real health. Every hour at my practice in London, the doorbell rings and a couple or an individual sits opposite me and pours out feelings. On one occasion, I had a thirty-one-year-old woman sobbing about her parents' divorce more than twenty years ago and why she couldn't find a lasting relationship. Even though she was a top-flight government adviser, it felt like I had a small child in the room as she looked up from her pile of crumpled tissues and asked, "Why did nobody think about me?"

Since the publication of my book, DIET FOR A NEW AMERICA, I have come into contact with an extraordinary array of dedicated people who are working diligently towards a truly healthy and sane world. I applaud these conscientious people and am encouraged by their efforts. One of these organizations is the Hippocrates Health Institute which has been turning people away from over-processed, health-destroying foods for decades, and I was pleased to accept their invitation to contribute a foreword to this book. Our culture has conditioned us away from contact with our spirits; taught us not to feel our bodies or respond to our emotions which has distracted us from heeding our innate wisdom. It has mechanized, trivialized and consumerized our basic human necessities, and reduced our most fundamental encounter with nature, the act of eating, into an act of death.

Death to the animals whose cooked corpses we euphemistically call steaks; death to our bodies through the disastrous health consequences of diets loaded with saturated fats and cholesterol and seriously depleted life force; and death to the environment which suffers such a heavy toll from the production of the standard diet.

We have been conditioned to think that only by eating meats, poultry, eggs and dairy products can we be well nourished. Yet, research is showing that these are the very foods that contribute so heavily to heart disease, cancer, diabetes, strokes and other degenerative diseases.

Today, more and more people are awakening from the hypnosis in which we have dutifully consumed the cooked corpses of animals. We are beginning to regain contact with the life force, and remembering that life is sacred. We are becoming sensitive enough to hear the signals coming from the wisdom of our own bodies. We are beginning to respect ourselves again, and to rejoin the web of life in gratitude and joy. We are realizing that life is good when we live in harmony with its laws.

Increasingly, people are becoming aware that eating can be a sacred communion, giving life to the spirit and health of the body. The time is passing in which it has actually been considered "natural" for people to eat a diet that is unhealthy, cruel to animals, and devastating to the life support systems of the biosphere. The time has arrived for people to be nourished body and soul by living foods, grown on living soils with respect for the earth and its creatures. The time has come for people to regain their health by eating a diet that is light, ethical and sustainable.

Thanks to groups such as the Hippocrates Health Institute, every morning there are more people who are venturing forth on the road to true harmony with nature's way. Each day they take further steps toward inner peace, and toward the happiness that each of us has always known deep inside ourselves was our responsibility to attain.

—John Robbins

Introduction

In his scientific writings, Holos Practice Reports, Dr. C. Norman Shealy has stated that our evolutionary ancestors ate only raw food selected by smell or taste. Further research indicated that natural raw or original food has the ability to trigger a satiety mechanism in one's body, effectively preventing overeating. Essentially, the body has received true nourishment and hunger is satisfied.

Various indications point to the fact that the human body was created to assimilate vegetation rather than meat. Human teeth, with their flat back molars and jaws that move both up and down, as well as sideways, may be an indication that we were not meant to be carnivorous. The same evidence exists in regard to our digestive tract which is about 36 feet long, totally unlike that of a carnivore, which is much shorter to allow for the quick passage of food and elimination of waste. The difference in the secretions of hydro-chloric acid to digest protein supports this distinction.

Obviously, we have deviated from nature's intended order regarding our nourishment. During the last century alone over 4,000 different additives have found their way into our food, which is also over-processed, over-cooked, denatured and even irradiated before being preserved and packaged. Our bodies find it difficult to recognize or assimilate what is being ingested. Most of these additive laden foods are incapable of regenerating the cells of the body.

The spraying of pesticides has become routine in the agricultural industry. John Robbins, in his book, "Diet For a New America" reveals shocking and disturbing information concerning the poisoning of our planet. His excellent work should sound an alarm to everyone that the accelerated use of poisonous chemicals is sheer madness. In one chapter he reveals that:

> "We produce pesticides today at a rate more than 13,000 time faster than we did only 35 years ago. Our environment and food chains are being inundated by a virtual avalanche of pesticides. What three decades ago took us six years to produce, we now produce every couple of hours."

> "It is hard for us to imagine how destructive these substances are. Pesticides are extraordinarily concentrated and powerful chemicals which have been intentionally developed to kill living creatures.

> In fact, some of them were originally developed to kill human beings. Phosgene, used today to produce chemical herbicides and in-secticides, was originally developed for use in chemical warfare, and was, in fact, the agent of almost all deaths due to poison gas in World War I."

Increasingly, energy that should be used for healing and rebuilding is being expended to process our body's waste. Our polluted world and diet with its assault on the immune system is the root cause of most illness. Our culture is accepting the illusion of health—we may think we eat well, and if we are uncertain of this fact, we often delude ourselves into believing that taking supplements will correct the deficiency. The average meal is mostly processed and cooked so that it is devoid of life and totally lacking in enzymes, the very essence of life. Such food cannot possibly nourish us except in the most minimal degree.

The result is malnutrition and the eventual breakdown of our immune system, our metabolic processes and our glandular functions. Toxic by-products and wastes from these chemical-laden foods accumulate in the body, while excess fats clog the arteries and veins. Excessive consumption; of proteins may cause tumors, create stones, or contribute to the enormous problem of excess weight.

This dreary picture could be discouraging were it not for the fact that encouraging changes are becoming evident, and people are realizing that health can be reclaimed through a change in lifestyle. By accepting responsibility for your health, perfect health, and nothing less, should be accepted. Simply stated, to have life in your body you must have life in your food.

We base our program on the premise that the following elements are essential to optimum health.

1. Wheatgrass chlorophyll is virtually identical to that derived from all rich green plants. This amazing plant contains complete protein, vitamins, minerals, and most importantly, oxygen, enzymes, hormones and phytonutrients and should be utilized throughout one's life.

2. Germinated and sprouted seeds and grains are essential to human health in providing easy digestibility and boundless maximum nutrition.

3. Raw alkalinizing juices on a daily basis are necessary to reverse the acidification process and to provide a full spectrum of nutrients.

4. An abundance of vegetables and judicious amount of fruit should be used to ensure a sound health-rebuilding program that will provide a buffer against our polluted environment.

5. Sunshine is the energy source of all life and plays a key role in strengthening our immunity.

6. Pure water and air are two foundations for our very existence.

7. Exercise is imperative and will speed the healing and rebuilding process by 40-50%.

8. Efficient digestive function and internal cleanliness provide an essential foundation on which to rebuild one's health. Proper food combining, the regular use of vegetable juices, fasting, and colon management techniques should not be overlooked as they provide the keys to life-long health.

9. Supplements derived only from whole foods such as algae, herbs, pollens, etc., not from fractionated forms or formulas, may be used as an adjunct but not as a substitute for healthful meals.

10. Integration of body/mind/spirit plays a central role in one's health. Understanding the mental impact of one's emotions on one's health clearly reveals the relevance of the mind/body connection. This underscores the importance of positive attitudes in one's pursuit of boundless health.

At this critical period in human history, we must face some challenging choices. However, we must also realize that this is not the end of the world; rather, it should be perceived as the beginning of a new era. We are fortunate to be living in an exciting period of history. Those who succeed, even thrive, during this time of drastic change will be those mature enough to recognize their responsibility to themselves, their planet, and their universe. Decades of experience in the health field has taught me that the responsible individual can and will flourish in this era.

The only fact that doesn't change is that change is a fact. People do not fit into neat categories, and we all need to experience the freedom that nourishes our infinite potential for growth and development in every facet of our lives. Experience benefits both the novice and the expert, and mistakes are often our most poignant and effective prod to make necessary "Changes". Experience teaches us to make wise choices, to weigh consequences and to savor the success that comes as a result of our enlightened judgment.

Our concepts are not far-fetched, and our vision of a flawless human existence does not exist in an imaginary Shangri-La. It is within our grasp if we would only surrender to the bountiful energy of life.

—Dr. Brian R. Clement

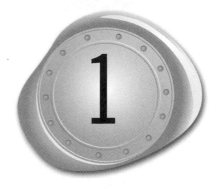

How Our Food Affects Our Life

A History of Leadership and Innovations

The Hippocrates Health Institute began in 1957 with the concept that the human body is a self-healing and self-rejuvenating organism, if given the proper tools and environment. Founded by Ann Wigmore and later co-founded by Viktoras Kulvinskas, the Institute's purpose was to research and implement research data in restoring the body to a state of optimum health through the use of live, enzyme-rich foods, wheatgrass and leafy green sprouts, along with alkalinizing juices to detoxify the body and quicken waste elimination. As the program evolved, its scope embraced daily exercises, a positive outlook on life, and an abiding faith that good will must prevail.

These powerful principles, based on a profound respect for all life, are not unique to our experience. The efforts of such pioneers, as Dr. Edmond

1

Bordeaux Szekely, who rediscovered these truths in his research into ancient civilizations and incorporated them into his own techniques, provided the foundation for other followers. Pioneers, such as Dr. Christine Nolfi, Dr. Norman Walker, and Herbert Shelton, to name just a few, are also honored here. The dedication of these early pioneers which include Ann Wigmore and Victorus Kulvinskas continues to benefit and influence today's health professionals. After decades, Hippocrates continues on the cutting edge as a natural health innovator. While recognizing that no one doctrine can dogmatically be claimed as having all the answers, we simply have endeavored to outline the basic knowledge we have gained through our considerable experience.

How We Have Deviated

In our present culture, it is apparent that we have deviated from living sensibly, especially where our nourishment is concerned. Much of our food intake comes in the form of fast foods, which merely appear to meet our needs but actually do not. They not only lack nourishment, but often contain harmful ingredients. For instance, let's take ice cream as an example.

In the past, ice cream was made of whole eggs, milk and sugar cranked out at home as an occasional treat. However, in today's synthetic era, we have a different story. This "fun food" is, in reality, a poison. Manufacturers are not required by law to list the additives used. Consequently, most ice creams contain some pretty surprising ingredients such as the following:

• •

DIETHYL GLYCOL—A cheap chemical used as an emulsifier instead of eggs, the same chemical used in anti-freeze and pain removers.

• •

PIPERONAL—Used instead of vanilla—a chemical used to kill lice.

• •

ALDEHYDE C 17—Used to flavor cherry ice cream it, is an inflammable liquid also used in aniline dyes, plastics and rubber.

• •

ETHYL ACETATE—Used to give a pineapple flavor, is also a leather cleaner—its vapors have been known to cause chronic organ damage.

• •

BUTYL ALDEHYDE—Used in nut flavored ice creams, is an ingredient in rubber cement

• •

ACRYL ACETATE—Used for banana flavor, is also a paint solvent.

• •

BENZYL ACETATE—Used for strawberry flavor, is a nitrate solvent.

Why Living and Raw Food—the Basics of Nourishment

With the spell of our illusions broken, we need to return to the natural way of eating and eliminate all chemicals from our food. Many ancient civilizations followed the ways of nature and knew the importance of eating live and raw natural foods, the basic source of nourishment. These basics are composed of raw, uncooked vegetables and fruits, germinated and sprouted grains, nuts and seeds, sprouted legumes, green sprouts grown on trays, alkalinizing juices, and some dehydrated and fermented foods.

Before we even examine the superior value of raw and living food we should explain exactly why we should not cook our food. During this apparently harmless process vital enzymes are destroyed, proteins are coagulated (making them very difficult to assimilate), and vitamins are mostly destroyed with the remainder changing into forms that are difficult for the body to utilize. Pesticides are restructured into even more toxic compounds, valuable oxygen is lost and free radicals are produced. Studies suggest that cooked proteins (coagulated) are up to 50% less likely to be utilized. Oxygen, enzymes, phytonutrients and hormones are consequently destroyed and acrylamides are created.

In addition, there is another danger in cooked foods that has special significance for our modern era with its overwhelming stresses on the human immune system making individuals increasingly vulnerable to a variety of diseases. Cooking food above a certain temperature (slightly under 200 degrees Fahrenheit) causes a pathogenic response in the body-leukocytosis—whereby white blood cells (leukocytes) are actually used to digest the food much as they would attack a foreign substance. In the last century, this was thought to be a normal part of the digestive process. However, Dr. Paul Kouchakoff, M.D. discovered in 1930 that consuming raw foods did not produce the same response. He also concluded that processing, before cooking, dramatically increased this pathological response.

Equally important to note is the absence of vital enzymes in cooked foods. The activity of life is enzyme activity, according to Dr. Edward Howell, a pioneer in this research. In his work he has identified up to 100,000 different enzymes functioning in the body. In the final analysis, he equates the health of individuals with their enzyme status. With these enzymes destroyed through cooking, our foods become enzyme deficient. Youthful bodies are capable of supplying additional enzymes needed to digest cooked foods, but this capability diminishes with age, causing indigestion and constipation in our older population. As one ages, it is more important than ever to eat a mainly raw diet.

A raw and living food diet is loaded with enzymes, crammed with vitamins and minerals, abundant in oxygen, complete with available proteins and is especially high in fiber. Furthermore, there is another life-giving response in the alkalinity of these foods. Most importantly, living foods, such as sprouts, which are still growing until the moment one eats them, provide us with a more subtle vitality due to the fact that the foods' bio-electrical forces are active. Kirlian photography has actually shown that the electrical energy surrounding a tray of wheatgrass is such that one's energy is enhanced by merely consuming them.

The abundance of oxygen in these foods should not be ignored. More and more studies reveal that oxygen deprivation within the body equals disease and death. Oxygenation of the blood stream is essential to the nourishment of all the cells in one's body. On a raw food diet, a continual supply of oxygen is fed into the system with extremely beneficial results. To reiterate, only living and raw foods with their alkaline effect on the body can reverse the acidification (aging, disease, and death) process caused by consumption of cooked and processed foods.

Definitive research on extending life spans has clearly proven that the consumption of high quality foods consumed in small amounts prolongs life. As always, the pharmaceutical industry is trying to create a pill which will help award us life extension. This pill will reduce caloric intake from food rather than to use common sense and educate people to eat less and get on the living food diet. Over the last half century there have been thousands of cases through the Life Transformation Program who arrived with a prognosis of demise and now, decades later, some in their 80's and 90's and even early 100's are flourishing contributors to the human race.

With these simple truths in mind, it is easy to see how harmony can be restored to the body through the use of fresh, raw and living foods. They nourish, cleanse and alkalinize the body by the combined action of their nutritional components, vitamins, minerals, amino acids (proteins), pure liquids, complex carbohydrates, fiber, enzymes, phytonutrients and hormones and oxygen.

• • •

Dr. Paul Kuchakoff &
Dr. Edward Howell
pioneered research that gave us
the scientific foundation which
proves humans were meant to eat
raw/living vegan diets

• • •

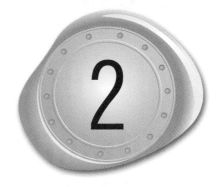

The Re-Emergence of An Old Truth

Supernutrition Through Germinating and Sprouting

In our work at the Hippocrates Institute, the use of raw and living foods has evolved into a new way of living and eating. We see a new relationship between food and life. Yet this relationship is not a new or novel concept, rather, it is a re-emergence of an ancient truth. The following are keys to this re-emerging system; the germinating and sprouting of foods, the use of grasses and leafy green vegetables, the importance of juices and the (careful) use of dehydrated and fermented foods.

Many ancient cultures knew the value of germinating and sprouting grains, seeds, legumes, beans and nuts. The use of sprouted seeds for food and medicine is more than twice as old as the Great Wall of China and was even noted in their historical records. Today more and more data is being compiled on the amazing nutritional value of sprouting. Research by

Dr. Jeffrey B. Land, professor and bio-chemist at the University of Puget Sound, has shown that 6 cups of sprouted lentils contain the full recommended daily allowance of protein (about 60 grams) in a fully digestible form. He then concluded that these could provide a significant portion of daily protein needs in a safe and inexpensive.

These living foods that are germinated and sprouted afford us the most concentrated natural sources of vitamins, chelated minerals, enzymes and amino acids (proteins in a digestible form). These also Contain abundant enzymes and bio-electrical energy, one important reason for their desirability. Pound for pound, lentils and bean sprouts contain as much protein as red meat, yet in a totally digestible form without the fat, cholesterol, hormones and antibiotics that are found in most present day meats.

Why this occurs bears some examination and explanation. Germination is the important process which results when seeds, grains, legumes and nuts are soaked in water for a period of time. Water removes certain metabolic inhibitors which are present to protect the seed from bacterial invasion and preserve it during its dormant state. Soaked seeds are more easily digested. During the germination process, the seed springs into life and becomes more available nutritionally for human needs. Inherent enzyme inhibitors, phytates (natural insecticides), oxalates, etc., present in every seed, nut or grain are removed through fermenting and before pre-digestion occurs. By this we mean that the starches are converted into simple sugars, proteins are broken down into amino acids, fats converted into soluble fatty acids and vitamins are created and enhanced. Germinating is the process employed to make many of the seeds and nut sauces at the Institute. For every one pound of seed, it will grow into eight to twelve pounds of superior food.

Sprouting carries this life-beginning process farther, resulting in a variety of living foods such as tray grown sprouts from sunflower seeds and pea seeds. Later on we will explain how to grow these green sprouts on trays. Several other sprouts are eaten before they develop any leaves.

Aside from the many health benefits from eating sprouts, these processes may present a solution to the growing problem of world hunger. By making inexpensive, abundant and highly nutritious foods like seeds, beans and grains even more healthful, sprouting is an ideal way to combat problems of dietary deficiency.

In our research at Hippocrates we have concluded that while there are virtually endless varieties of foods that can be sprouted, certain categories of the most beneficial sprouts have evolved which provide for very different types of utilization by the body. As the following partial chart suggests, Groups 1 and 2 are for cleansing and rebuilding the body, while Groups 3 and 4 provide maximum energy and endurance and are jokingly referred to as the "macho sprouts". Group 5 is for the re-mineralization of the body due to the high mineral content of these unique beans which must be sprouted with the complete absence of sunlight stimulation to provide this vital effect. Group 6 is also unique, due to its internal gentle healing quality, not unlike that of a nurturing parent versus the dramatic healing effect of the chlorophyll-rich, tray-grown green sprouts like wheatgrass, sunflower and green pea. Each of these has a unique quality and should be considered in your daily dietary choices. Sprouts are not only economical, practical and magnificent givers of life and health, but are perfect foods for environmental purposes. Indeed they are the food for generations to come.

Tray Greens

Also integral to your program is the green sprouts of sunflower and green pea seeds. These are sprouted, and then planted in soil on trays, similar to wheatgrass. Basically, this amounts to indoor gardening. These tray-grown sprouts are equally rich in chlorophyll and nutrients. With the wheatgrass they comprise a major portion of the "living food" at the Institute. They are eaten in salads shortly after harvesting and are juiced for "green drinks" which are consumed twice daily on your program. A green drink consists of a variety of green vegetable juices and at least 50% should be green sprout juice. Not only do these drinks alkalinize the system but they provide immediate, highest quality, full spectrum nutrition to the body. One is simply not on the Hippocrates Diet unless consuming at least two of these drinks a day.

Both the wheatgrass and the sprout greens are economical and easy to grow. To begin, you will need ordinary topsoil combined with 50% peat moss—both readily available at any nursery. As you progress, you will be producing the highest quality compost from discarded root mats and your soil will improve continually. Additionally, you will be partaking in a soil regeneration program, returning to the earth and recycling what was taken out.

You will need trays to hold the soil. We use planting trays with drainage. One tray is needed to hold the soil and seeds for planting, and another as a cover to hold in the moisture. If you want to have one tray of wheatgrass every day, you will need about 16 trays in all. For the greens you may use as many or fewer, depending on your needs. By experimenting with different amounts you will eventually find the right number of trays you to need to plant.

To store the soil and peat moss mixture, an empty trash container might suffice. If you plan to compost the used root mats, you will need another such container with holes drilled every four inches round for air circulation. More information on composting will follow.

To plant wheatgrass, soak one cup of whole winter wheat seeds for 8 hours in a lot of water. Then sprout for another 8 hours with the jar upside down in a dish drainer. Rinse at last two times in warm water to prevent drying out. Then spread a one inch layer of soil over the tray, being careful not to let the seeds spill in the trough. Try not to let the seeds pile on top of one another. Sunflower and peas are planted more densely than wheat because their root systems are not as strong. Water thoroughly but do not over water. You can tell if you have over watered if you see it standing in the gutter. Next, place the cover and leave it for three days or until the lid starts to lift as a result of the sprouts pushing it up. At that point uncover and water thoroughly and place in a bright spot but not in direct sunlight. Water once a day along the trough. Your plants will be mature enough to use in a total of seven days, depending on the weather and climate.

The procedure for growing tray-grown sprouts of sunflower and buckwheat is similar. When purchasing your seeds be sure to buy seeds with their hulls left on and purchase organically grown or biologically grown seeds. For each tray soak 1½ cups sunflower and ¾ sup dry buckwheat seeds in quart jars filled with water. The amount of water you will need is one full quart for the sunflower and ½ quart for the peas. Soak for eight hours, then drain the seeds and allow them to sprout for 8 to 12 hours. Plant them in the same way as wheatgrass.

To compost the soil from the tray after harvesting the sprouts you break the root mats apart and place them in a plastic garbage can with holes drilled every four inches. Cover the can and continue to add layers of mats and vegetable scraps from the kitchen, especially the pulp from the juicer, until the can is full. In about three months, the soil inside will be ready to use for planting. To use this recycled soil at 25% peatmoss for improved moisture retention.

The Value of Juices

Fresh juices are another key to the Hippocrates program. The extracted juices from fresh vegetables, and tray-grown sprouts allow us to gain all the benefits and outstanding nutritional qualities in an easily assimilated form. These are digested immediately and begin cleansing and healing long before the same whole foods begins to work. In addition, whole foods use up valuable energy because of the prolonged digestion process which can be applied in healing.

Juicing is not the same thing as blending or even liquefying. A blender makes a fruit or vegetable appear liquefied, whereas a juicer extracts only the liquid (nutrition), leaving the cellulose or fiber behind. At Hippocrates, we use several juicers for preparing fresh juices. Auger presses are excellent machines. They juice greens and grass; a job that the high speed machines cannot do efficiently. A Norwalk press can also be used to extract leafy green juice.

A popular breakfast at the Institute is watermelon juice made with any of the mentioned juicers. During juicing we include the rind and seeds. This juice is excellent for the kidneys and bladder and it functions beautifully as a diuretic. By utilizing the whole food, the sugar content is reduced and there is additional protein as well as vitamins A, B and C and chlorophyll.

As mentioned before, the "green drinks" on our living food program are vital to health and well-being. These are made from juiced sunflower and peagreen sprouts and vegetables such as cucumber, celery, parsley, watercress, edible weeds, etc. All are juiced in a slow turning juicer like the wheatgrass juicer. What gives these drinks their healing qualities is that they are made with the indoor, tray-grown sprouts. These are nutritionally packed "living foods" and the other vegetable juices are merely added for flavor. We recommend that everyone drink at least two eight ounce glasses of "green drink" per day. These "green drinks" are an exceptional source of chlorophyll with its attendant oxygen. They can also supply the complete pre-digested protein needed each day (about 25 grams). Another factor about these juices we wish to emphasize is their desired alkalinizing effect upon the body.

Sprouting

Germinating a bean, seed, nut, legume or grain is a beautifully simple procedure. Basically all that is needed is a jar, some seeds and water. To germinate for sauces, etc., just soak the seeds or nuts the required time in the purest water available. Be sure to rinse well to remove all inhibitors before preparing sauces, seed milks, etc. The seeds or nuts are now ready to be made into delicious dressings, sauces or seed and nut loaves. One can learn how to prepare these in our recipe books.

Sprouting requires a few more simple steps. First, be aware that soaking time varies according to the size of the seed. All small seeds similar to alfalfa, radish, red clover, sesame, cabbage, mustard, etc. can be soaked for 4 to 6 hours. Larger nuts and beans like almonds, filberts, Brazil nuts, pinto, chickpeas, etc. can be soaked for 10 to 12 hours. However, climate, season and temperature play a significant role as in warmer times soaking is greatly reduced. We must reiterate, for mung and aduki beans to realize their full potential as life-givers to the body, they must be sprouted in darkness, recreating the pattern nature created for them.

To begin, you will need some wide mouth jars, some plastic screen mesh, a rubber band to secure the mesh to the top of the jar, and, of course, the seeds. People who are away from home daily will find automatic sprouters are a useful piece of equipment. For traveling, sprouting can be accomplished in sprouting bags.

After soaking the appropriate time, pour off the soak water and rinse well. Turn the jar upside down to let it drain. Use a dish drainer to hold the jar at an angle. Then continue to rinse the sprouts morning and evening to keep them from drying out. It is important to keep them moist, warm and well-drained. Room temperature is ideal—in warmer climates they will grow more quickly with a greater chance to spoil. So rinse them more often in warmer area.

Between rinsing, place the jars upside down at a 45 degree angle to allow for drainage and circulation. When they are ready you will want to remove the hulls of such seeds as alfalfa, fenugreek, cabbage, mung, aduki and radish. Others, such as the grains, hulled sunflower seeds, sesame seeds, lentils and chickpeas can be eaten as they are. To remove hulls, place the sprouts in the sink or a large pan and fill with water. Then carefully stir the sprouts to loosen the hulls and brush the hulls aside. Next, carefully lift the floating sprouts out of the water so as not to disturb the hulls which are floating along the sides or sunk to the bottom. Place the hulled sprouts in a colander to drain. Sprouts will keep in the refrigerator for about a week, but the quicker you eat them the richer they are in nutrients.

Some words about sprouts are in order. Small seeds do gradually increase in weight and volume after sprouting, so don't overfill the jar. These may be set in direct light for a few days to green their leaves.

Wheatgrass—The Green Miracle

Another key to Hippocrates' success has been wheatgrass, a miraculous food that is now widely recognized as a health builder and restorative. This truth is also not a new concept. Over 50 million years ago, the emergence of the grasses caused a major reorganization of the animal world and those that could utilize its nourishing qualities thrived. Though we humans do not have the ability to process large quantities of these grass fibers, current research is showing that chlorophyll extract (juice) is an excellent phytonutrient healer.

Wheatgrass juice is one of nature's richest sources of vitamins A, C and E and contains all of the known mineral elements. It is rich in calcium, phosphorous, iron, potassium, sulphur, sodium, cobalt and zinc. According to recent research, the grasses are exceptionally high in B vitamins, especially vitamin B-17 (laetrile). Wheatgrass contains chlorophyll, a substance that is referred to as nature's great healer. Chlorophyll produces an unfavorable environment for bacterial growth in the body and helps purify the liver, builds a clean bloodstream and aids in proper digestion, as well as helping to balance the blood sugar. Wheatgrass is a complete protein.

Because wheatgrass is a powerful cleanser, it may cause nausea in some people soon after ingestion. This is merely a reaction to the release of toxins within the system. Start with small quantities, one ounce or so and gradually increase the intake to four ounces. By implanting Wheatgrass juice directly into the colon, it is used as part of a sound colon cleansing program, a process we will describe in detail later.

Once juiced, wheatgrass is not stable and tends to go bad quickly so it is best to use it immediately or within 15 minutes. However, cut grass will store for a week or so in the refrigerator in plastic containers, (bags, etc.). Frozen wheatgrass juice will keep for some time, but is not effective like freshly made juice, containing only a shadow of its whole benefit.

Dehydrated and Fermented Foods

Another method we employ is dehydration, the bridge from cooked to raw foods. This method of drying fruits, vegetables, nut-and-seed mixtures opens a door to a whole new world of healthy nutritious and delicious eating. Dehydrators are readily available today and while some vitamin and enzyme breakdown occurs during this process, it is still much preferred to cooking. We should mention that you must purchase the highest quality organic produce available, making certain it is fresh and fully ripe.

Fruit has long been thought of as the ultimate food by many on health quests. However, we have observed that while small amounts of fruit in the daily diet are usually fine, an all fruit, or mostly fruit diet is over-stimulating and aggravating to certain illnesses. In cases of advanced disease no fruit should be consumed. Such a diet is too rich in sugar to be used so extensively in our modern world. Of course, for blood sugar, cancer, yeast and microbial problems even a small amount is unacceptable. Therefore, at the Institute we recommend less fruit and more vegetables.

Fermented foods are also controversial in their benefits. For many years we advocated a wide variety of fermented foods and drinks for all people, but we noticed that they sometimes caused adverse reactions. Fermented drinks like Rejuvelac and fermented seed cheeses and nut loaves were found to harbor some unfriendly bacteria. For most health seekers, occasional raw sauerkraut is enough.

In rounding out our dietary program, I wish to clarify a few points. While a 100% raw food diet is ideal, many of us need to function in a toxic, lower vibrational world. In order to facilitate this we have found that, unless serious health problems exist, a diet of 80% raw and living food and 20% cooked food is acceptable. Steamed vegetables, high-performance grains like quinoa, amaranth and the alkaline millet, baked squashes and yams are good nutritional choices. Also, with the increasing evidence that serious disease results from an excess of three basics—proteins, fats and sugars—we firmly recommend, even on a living food diet, that proportions should be as follows by weight: 5% proteins from algae, germinated or sprouted seeds and nuts; 5% fats from whole foods like avocado, sprouts, nuts & seeds with the major portion of the food, 90% coming from complex carbohydrates, such as sprouts, greens and raw vegetables with occasional fruits.

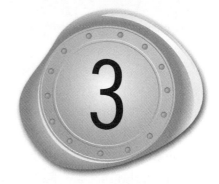

Optimum Assimilation and Digestion

Proper Food Combining

As important as it is to know which foods and drinks to choose, it is just as important to know how to combine food properly. While one mixture of foods aids digestion, another can create the reverse situation. While most live foods combine well with each other because of their composition, there are a few rules which should be followed:

First, do not drink liquids with meals as they will dilute the gastric secretions, making digestion more difficult. Second, fruits and vegetables do not mix well. They are better eaten at separate meals, or one should wait at least two hours after eating fruit to eat vegetables. Sprouts are included in the vegetable category, as is wheatgrass. When eating a fruit dessert, also wait for at least two hours after the main course.

When eating fruit meals or single fruits, try to make combinations of acid fruits with other acid fruits, subacid with subacid and sweet fruits together with other sweet or dried fruits, rather than mixing the 3 groups indiscriminately. Each of the groups of fruits has a different water and sugar content, and they are more easily digested when eaten with similar fruits. It is also important to eat melons by themselves. Melons are one of the most quickly and easily digested foods. When combined with other fruits as in a fruit salad, their digestion is delayed by the more slowly digested fruits and this can cause fermentation. Avocados are the only exception to the fruit/vegetable rule. They are easily combined with either fruits or vegetables, making them a truly versatile and nourishing food.

Eliminative Health

For proper assimilation and digestion we need to maintain a healthy colon. The average person is preoccupied with the cleanliness of his home, car, etc., and gives little thought to his internal state of cleanliness. Thus, millions of people have colons that are impacted with toxic waste. Laxatives and other over-the-counter remedies have become big business, with colon cancer emerging as the number two cancer killer in this nation.

The colon's main function is to eliminate unusable portions of food and other metabolic waste from the body. During the final phase of digestion, liquids and some minerals are removed from the food and the colon and then are ready to be recycled. When the colon is clean and functioning normally, we experience a state of wellness, and when it is congested and twisted out of shape, it can cause problems in other parts of the body. A badly impacted colon can be carrying unwanted fecal matter. Even though a person may have a daily bowel movement, there may still be several days' worth (even up to a week's worth) of waste inside the colon. This provides a breeding ground for unfriendly bacteria which can cause a multitude of problems, including headaches, flatulence, indigestion, colitis, bowel cancer and other physical disorders. When these wastes have accumulated in the colon the peristaltic becomes weak and sluggish, causing constipation. These accumulations tend to harden in the pockets of the colon walls. This hardened material obstructs the peristalsis (the natural muscular contraction of the bowel) and more and more buildup occurs. This then interferes with final absorption and digestion, so that instead of absorbing nutrients; the undigested food putrefies, creating toxic conditions.

The first step necessary in cleansing the colon is the use of enemas and, occasionally, colonics. Then, use chlorophyll (made from wheatgrass or algae) implants, and change your diet to living foods. We have found through years of research with our guests that instead of harming the electrolyte balance in the colon, enemas with implants actually restore a better balance. After taking a room temperature distilled water enema, this is the way to take a high wheatgrass implant. Fill the enema bag with at least four ounces of fresh undiluted juice. Proceed with the implant using the ordinary enema procedure. Then remove the catheter and remain lying down. Retain the implant for 15-20 minutes before expelling it.

Other rules for colon management are common sense and, therefore, oftentimes overlooked. Heeding natures call to eliminate is extremely important, especially the first thing in the morning when bowel functions have been active all night. Regular exercise is also important, and the lack of exercise immediately after eating because the process of digestion requires a great deal of energy.

Finally, one small device which we use to great advantage is a foot stool, platform or box to go under both feet, when seated on the toilet. By raising the feet off the ground, we are in a squatting position which is really our natural position encouraging better elimination, and the design of the modern toilet may actually contribute to constipation problems.

Fasting

Equally important is the role of fasting as a part of life. Throughout history, fasting has been recognized as one of the best methods to eliminate toxic accumulations from the system. While most natural health proponents accept fasting, there are two distinct schools of thought and some convincing arguments are made on each side of the controversy.

One group strongly supports water fasting as the correct way to fast, arguing that taking of any type of liquid nourishment cannot be considered a true fast. On the other hand, a different school suggests that fasting with vegetable and fruit juices brings far better results, without the severe reactions that often accompany lengthy periods of food deprivation.

At the Institute, we subscribe to this latter point of view, and our extensive experience in our work has convinced us that this is the best course to follow. Severe reactions may attend a water fast which can cause unnecessary stress on the organs of elimination. Drinking water only greatly accelerates the cleansing process causing massive amounts of toxins to be released from the body. Juice fasting, while just as effective, evinces less trauma and discomfort. More importantly, on a juice fast one is nourished and strengthened instead of being depleted and weakened.

Anyone planning to try a first-time fast should consult a health professional who can help should difficult cleansing reactions occur.

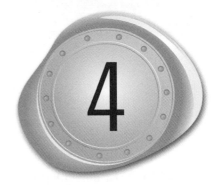

Expanding The Parameters of Health

In addition to a more correct relationship of food to life, our research at the Institute has verified the need to expand the parameters of healthful living to include certain other basics. Who will deny the importance of sunlight, air and water in a full, natural life? Yet, in today's polluted environment the search for these elements, which are so necessary, has become problematical.

Attention must also be paid to detoxifying the larger environment, beginning with one's home and workplace. Clothing must be re-examined. Our diet and approach to life represents a health restoring lifestyle that makes it imperative to break away from the manipulative systems of the special interests that dominate our world today. Fast foods, drugs, chemicals, additives and preservatives should be assiduously avoided.

Sunlight, Air and Water

The vital importance of sunlight cannot be overemphasized in any healthful approach to life. Ancient peoples revered the sun as life-giver and healer. In current thinking, however, the sun is depicted as purely destructive and contributes to aging.

Yet there is scientific body of evidence that suggest the modern diet has actually created the negative conditions that sunlight only accelerates. At the Institute we favor this latter opinion and advise moderate sun exposure, in the morning or evening, which helps healing by lowering blood pressure, establishing a better blood sugar balance, aiding digestion and strengthening the immune system. The absorption of vitamin D from the sun's rays helps to build strong bones and prevent disorders.

Today there is increasing evidence that most incandescent bulbs and fluorescent tubes have a potentially harmful effect on the human system. Again there are measures we can take to alter these factors in our favor. Science has recognized for some time that light and color affect our whole being. One breakthrough in this type of research was made by F. Jacobsen, M.D. and Norman Rosenthal, M.D. which they named "Seasonal Affective Disorder and the Use of Light as an Anti-Depressant", conducted under the auspices of the National Institute of Mental Health in Bethesda, Maryland.

The original pioneer in this field was Dr. John Ott, who researched extensively the effects of artificial and natural light on the human system. Basically, he determined that a lack of sunlight (full spectrum light) in seasonal periods caused a wide range of mental and emotional problems—from lethargy to full-blown depression—in a wide segment of the population.

He further determined that the sun's rays play a major role in the state of our physical health, especially the immune response. The top echelon of science today is validating these conclusions.

Rouleau is a complex modern malady found in the bloodstream of people who operate computers and other electronics. Basically, this is a "bending" of the blood cells, causing the cells to coagulate and contort their shape, creating massive vulnerabilities and potential disease. This condition is caused by the harmful light frequencies and electronic vibrations emitted from these terminals. Also of serious concern here are possible links to eye problems, miscarriages and birth defects. Swedish studies have reported significantly higher rates of birth defects in babies born to women who work regularly at video display terminals during their pregnancies. The only antidote would be the use of full spectrum lighting, applied directly over the operator during terminal use and certain shielding materials covering the screen. Television viewers should sit at least 6 feet away from the screen and even farther would be better.

There is a profusion of health complications brewing from modern inventions that we have not been alerted to as yet. Beside the evident fact that "winter blues" and seasonal ups-and-downs are universally felt, we have somehow neglected to understand the importance of all of the elements in nature. When living in an inclement climate, one should rely on either full spectrum lighting or UV (ultra-violet frequencies included) lights which are less expensive. These should be everywhere in your home; from the light next to your chair to those in your bathroom. They are becoming more available all the time through health food stores, specialty outlets, and on the internet.

The quality of the air we breathe is of great importance to a healthy life. Proper breathing cannot be overemphasized. While we can touch only superficially upon this serious subject, it is important to state how vital it is to breathe deeply in order to oxygenate the blood stream if one is to be truly healthy. Most people simply do not breathe deeply enough. The result of this is the bloodstream becomes oxygen deficient, leading to all types of physical including brain function problems.

One of the best ways to oxygenate the blood stream is through vigorous exercise. That is why our exercise program is such an important part of our courses. However, we do start out slowly because so many of our guests have not exercised regularly prior to visiting the Institute. The benefits do accrue rather quickly though, and this is due to the greatly increased oxygenation.

The quality of the air in one's environment is of equal importance, especially in view of the fact that the skin, the largest organ in the body, also absorbs oxygen. Wearing synthetic clothing for extended periods may be quite harmful because the skin must breathe. Regardless of where one lives, air pollution is becoming a serious problem. Having a complete indoor garden of wheatgrass, tray-grown sprouts and houseplants, helps to oxygenate indoor air. There are some quality air treatment systems on the market today that bear investigation. We can provide information on these if you write to us.

Pure water is another basic need. Water pollution has become a worldwide problem and we should take special precautions with the water we use. While there are many sophisticated water filter and purifiers on the market today for drinking purposes, we recommend distilled water, either processed at home or purchased in glass containers. There are so many dangerous substances in our water at this time that distillation seems to make the most sense. Unlike some past thinking on this, distilled water does not leach minerals from the body. Granted, distilled water is unstructured, which basically means its molecular structure is in need of "organizing" before the body can utilize it. However, exposure to sunlight for ½ hour can change this. Actually, on a living food diet, the most important source of structure, distilled water is in the food and raw juice itself, the highest quality and greatest quantity being found in sprouts. One other choice is distilled structured water which not only organizes the H2O molecules; it creates the strongest anti-oxidant effect in your cells fighting against disease.

Detoxify Your Home

For a healthy life we need to consider the environment. There is a growing awareness of the threat of indoor air pollution. Insecticides, formaldehyde, asbestos, radon gas, lead, tobacco smoke, etc. pose a serious threat in our energy-efficient, weather tight and inadequately ventilated homes. According to High Kaufman, hazardous waste expert at the Environmental Protection Agency, "We're just beginning to identify the problem of indoor air pollution, but everywhere we look it is worse than be expected".

Practically any enclosed building can become the source of dangerous contaminants due to the buildup of volatile chemical concentrations exuded from plastics and solvents. The combustible particulates from heating plants and tobacco, which give off nitrogen dioxide, carbon monoxide and hydrocarbons, provide and ideal setting for the cultivation of fungi, nematodes and bacteria that may cause respiratory ailments such as legionnaire's disease, among others.

According to the Consumer Product Safety Commission, manufactured particle board, plywood, carpet backing, furniture, permanent press clothing and insulated materials emit poisonous formaldehyde gases that can progress to more serious conditions. A recent study of 164 mobile homes, in four randomly selected trailer parks, revealed that more than half of them exceeded what are considered safe levels of formaldehyde concentrations.

Especially dangerous is urea-formaldehyde foam insulation. Some research has indicated a definite link to crib deaths. If you suspect such a problem in your home, you can obtain a "dosimeter" to measure concentration of formaldehyde. The Environment Protection Agency may be able to provide information on this matter.

Another widespread and dangerous indoor pollutant is radon gas, a radioactive substance emitted from the earth's crust from uranium deposits found in much of inhabited earth. Exposure can occur, unknowingly, through such simple activities as using a washing machine or taking a hot shower. Here again, testing should be available in your area. Homeowners can minimize gas seepage into cellars by sealing off all masonry cracks and by providing adequate ventilation in living areas.

Another source of indoor pollution that should not be forgotten is cigarette smoke. British researchers have recently discovered that urine samples of 85% of the non-smokers tested contained measurable levels of tobacco substances even though some of these individuals did not believe that they were being subjected to second-hand smoke.

Carbon monoxide is another killer that may be stalking a weather-tight home. Poorly ventilated furnaces, gas dryers and unvented kerosene heaters are all possible sources of carbon monoxide poisoning. Also, prolonged exposure to common Household chemicals found in various cleaners, soaps, disinfectants, pesticides, paint thinners and all volatile substances should be avoided.

For many years the approved treatment for termite infestation has been the use of chlordane. However, research now has shown that this poison does not break down, as was previously thought, and dangerous contamination may continue indefinitely. There have been many cases where homes have actually been abandoned because heating ducts were contaminated with this deadly substance.

This list could go on and on. Such indoor environment hazards may seem to be beyond one's control, but to be aware of possible dangers allows us to explore safer options and to take corrective measures. Also, through ignorance, we may further add dangerous pollutants to our home environment. By being aware of these hazards, we are able to avoid much pain and grief.

Clothing

Our clothing may also be potentially hazardous to our health. This area has yet to be investigated fully. Accumulating data indicates that synthetic fabrics do affect our health. The advent of these fibers has imperiled many super-sensitive people by the wide-spread and unregulated use of chemical agents, flame retardants, solvents, acid and dyes. These are used to treat both natural and synthetic fabrics. Of all the chemical processes involved, the flame retardants have been the most widely publicized, and these have been found to be both mutagenic and carcinogenic in research.

Of equal danger is vinyl chloride, a highly toxic chemical known to be carcinogenic in humans. It is used frequently in synthetic fabrics, especially in fake furs and wigs. This is extremely dangerous where wigs are concerned, due to the high permeability of the scalp.

For all these reasons, not to mention the larger negative impact on the environment from chemical wastes created by these synthetics, we recommend only natural fibers—cotton, linen, wool, flax, hemp and all organic. Because of their breathability, these fibers are the most comfortable.

Caring for clothing is important. As much as possible, try to wash your clothing in a biodegradable product and avoid spot removers, pre-washing treatments and bleach. The residues they leave behind may produce skin irritations and allergic reactions, and these products have a negative impact on the environment as well. Dry cleaning should be used as little as possible unless green. With garments that must have this process, let them air outdoors for about a week so that most of the fumes can be dispersed.

Planetary Wellness

The program that we evolved at the Institute is a completely integrated system. The foods we choose and those we grow are returned to the earth through composting. Our every aim here is to live healthfully and in complete harmony with the earth. Living within this framework helps to protect us from the machinations and manipulations of special interests. This program will give you total control of your dietary choices, leading to full responsibility for your own health. This approach, beginning on an individual level and expanding outward, can lead to planetary harmony as well.

Over our lives we have been discouraged from living with Passion. Layers of unwanted involvements weigh heavily on us and diminish our spirits. When this spark is gone we cannot appreciate life and live with the joy and freedom which is our birthright. This is why one must make their main objective to fulfill themselves through an impassioned focus on those things that give you the most joy.

Those people who feel out of touch with themselves spew their discontent all over the planet creating everything from unsafe energy sources to piles of rubble as they discard whatever they wish out the windows of their cars, off the sides of their boats and in the garbage cans in front of their homes and businesses. Trained by a market-based culture we are avid consumers who do not think about tomorrow and, more importantly, do not care about today. This destructive activity has led us into a disease causing environment filled with our discards, and as nature always will, she is trying to let us know that we must stop. Disease rates are growing, multiplying and mutating. Each year there are hundreds of new symptoms and disorders that cannot be categorized under the traditional health criteria. We have observed the recipients of catastrophic disease becoming younger and younger as time passes. You must stand strong and think and act independently so that you are a contributor to yours and others advancement rather than just one more burden on the planet.

Make sure that all you think and do is in harmony with your deepest heartfelt desires. This will assure that your future affords the potential to live disease free and successfully enriched.

• • •

**You must stand strong,
think and act independently,
so that you are a contributor
to yours and others
advancement, rather
than just one more burden
upon the future of the planet.**

• • •

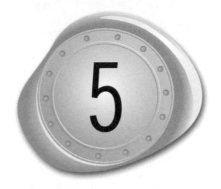

The Exercise
Imperative

Fitness today is largely considered an integral part of life. Indeed, fitness is big business with improving techniques, medical research in this area, and a wide assortment of fitness equipment. At the Institute, we strive for a full understanding of the underlying principles governing our physical response to exercise, and how these responses enable the body to become totally well. Most individuals equate exercise only with weight control, body contouring, flexibility and muscular strength. Actually, these desired results are more cosmetic and are less important than the major benefits that affect the individual internally.

The vascular system, lymphatic system, circulatory system, digestive system, immune system and respiratory system are profoundly dependent upon physical activity for their efficient functioning. On an emotional level, we benefit immensely through a reduction of stress, anxiety, lethargy and depression.

Exercise generally fits into two distinct categories: those that stretch the muscles and those that strengthen them. Both movements are necessary to achieve optimum fitness. We have found that a program of daily stretching exercises promotes optimum cleansing of the body's tissues. A condition of stagnation and congestion is the prime contributor of most degenerative physical problems. Stretching exercises best enable these congealed masses of toxic residues to become dislodged and eliminated.

One of the worst things we do to ourselves in not to exercise. The buildup of bodily wastes becomes increasingly toxic, so we need vigorous daily exercise; thus the bloodstream can move through the muscles forcefully, carrying away these toxic residues.

Furthermore, exercise that is sufficiently vigorous oxygenates the blood, enhancing this cleansing process. The lymphatic fluid, so vital to the breakup of accumulated wastes surrounding the cells, is also activated. Rebounders or mini-trampolines are helpful in this respect. Gentle bouncing for about five minutes daily will enable the lymph fluids to wash back and forth over the cells, loosening waste residues so that they can be carried away in the blood stream. With the blood stream as the sanitation department of the body, we can keep it in top form by exercising daily.

The other type of exercise we should include is the type that strengthens or contracts the muscles. Resistance exercise, swimming and weight training fall into this category. This type of workout builds strength and promotes a healthy cardiovascular system. Vigorous aerobic exercise combined with resistance exercise is a strong preventative of osteoporosis, because any impact on the skeletal system causes more calcium to be absorbed into the bones to compensate for the stress.

There are close to 700 muscles in the human body. If muscles are not exercised they atrophy. Just as a variety of foods provides the best balance of nutriments, so do many different types of activities give our complicated muscular structure the workout each muscle requires to maintain a high degree of fitness.

There are so many enjoyable activities to choose from as a form of exercise such as swimming, walking, rowing, biking, dancing, running, weight training, aerobics, volleyball, golf, tennis, shuffleboard, bowling and many other sports. Regardless of your age, you can find an appropriate activity that will strengthen your heart and oxygenate your bloodstream.

Exercise, self-esteem, diet and happiness will bring a person to the apex of health. We should all aspire to a full and meaningful life experience. As we help the individuals who participate in our program to improve their perspective and activate their dreams, we know that there are truly no boundaries or limits to what anyone can accomplish. Happiness and fulfillment is always within reach of everyone who follows nature's magnificent methods.

• • •

**Less than five percent
of the developed world's
population exercise adequately.**

• • •

6

Body/Mind/Spirit/ Unfolding Into Wellness

In our work of teaching how one may attain total health, we employ several other techniques quite successfully. Massage and more aggressive body work, such as deep muscle and shiatsu, have often proven effective. Massage affects every part of the body—glands, organs, tissues, muscles, nerves, circulation, lymph, etc. Not only does it stimulate elimination of poisons, but it also calms the mind and gives immediate emotional gratification. Steam baths and hot tub baths, as well as saunas, are also employed effectively. We have found that steam baths clean the water organs such as kidneys and lungs, while the sauna works on the fat organs, specifically the liver and gallbladder. The whirlpool gives relaxing warmth to the body and benefits the nerve tissue lymph and bones.

Reflexology may be another useful tool in self-healing, and acupuncture, Nucca or cranial reconstruction may accelerate the healing process. There is no reason to limit oneself in exploring these and many other options.

Prayer, meditation and visualization techniques are also an integral phase of our work, and we have found those techniques pioneered by Bernie Siegal, Norman Cousins, Louise Hay, Dr. Larry Doussey and Dr. Simonton of equal value.

Through the conscious application of these methods, an improvement in the body/mind/spirit complex occurs naturally when combined with a living food diet. Under ideal circumstances, the total energy available to us is divided equally into 3 areas: 1/3 in the physical area (governing food, fear, sex, etc.), 1/3 in the emotional area (governing understanding of self and others), and the remaining 1/3 in the mental/spiritual area (governing universality).

Today 91% of our energy is locked into the physical level; 8% operates in the emotional area; and less than 1% of our total energy ever reaches the mental/spiritual level of self-preservation and the satisfaction of pure physical desires. However, on a living food diet, amplified by other correct approaches to "Right Living" we can transcend these earth-bound tendencies and develop our highest mental and spiritual nature.

• • •

**Living food
together with
strengthening and
stimulation of the body,
positive thought and
spiritual application
creates
healthy and happy lives**

• • •

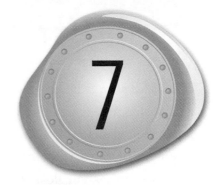

Modern Dilemmas

Addictions

Another concern existing today that threatens the integrity of humanity is the scourge of addictions and drug abuse. Addiction to alcohol, smoking, food, drugs, sugar, gambling, caffeine, television, pornography, fanatic ideology and similar mental aberrations are causing untold suffering. Because many individuals find it difficult to cope with daily stresses they try to escape momentarily by using various destructive tools. The crashing return back to reality leads to an ever escalating dependence on these mind-altering substances. Our occupation with escapism clouds our view and prevents us from living up to our highest potential. A drunken stupor or an elusive high are the by-products of helplessness, fear and self-doubt. When over one-half of our children at age 12 have partaken of some type of drug or alcohol, we had better start seeking solutions to this widespread and vexing issue.

The person using extremely addictive drugs requires professional help. Rehabilitation can be costly and drawn out, but addicts have no other choice if their lives are to be saved. However, the road back can be hastened with a cleansing and nourishing live food diet that will help strengthen and repair drug damaged bodies.

For smokers, we recommend certain stop-smoking programs as being effective choices. For alcohol and other drug addiction, we feel well established organizations such as rehab centers around the world should be the first stop. After going through a professional detoxification program, the next natural step should be a Life Transformation Program such as ours, where one will learn a balanced, natural lifestyle which will reinforce one's emotional strengths and gratify one's nutritional needs. This helps to promote balance and lessen the need for depressants or stimulants.

Those with sugar and caffeine addictions do quite well on our program as the body is so quickly satisfied and nourished, especially with the alkalinizing green drinks, that much of the root cause of the addiction is wiped away.

We view all things in life in a very simple fashion. There are only a few basic principles that govern creation. One is the value we place in ourself. To experience health and to reach our mental, emotional and spiritual goals, we should make wise choices in every area of life, from the type of food we consume, to how we deal with others, as well as how we treat our environment.

No one can be totally independent. We all need each other, and, by being a shining example of buoyant health, we can inspire and motivate others to transform their diseased bodies into bodies expressing boundless health. This wonderful transformation on a personal level continues to benefit and influence others, constantly enlarging in scope, till it eventually transforms the entire world.

Hypoglycemia

Fifty years ago, hypoglycemia was virtually unknown to the majority of health-care professionals. When people world complain of emotional swings, unnatural cravings, fatigue and physical upset, most medical doctors would refer them to a psychiatrist or psychologist. I have personally worked with several hundred people who had been down this deceptive and confusing road when their only real problem was the lack of regulated natural blood sugars. With the blood sugar level too low, the body's pancreas will constantly "lash out" in search of any sugars to try to bring this level up to normal. Most people still do not know that unless one is born with diabetes, the first stage of that disease is usually hypoglycemia. Everyone who now has diabetes has first suffered from a hypoglycemic condition. Consequently, this disease should be given serious attention.

Through my work with thousands of people, I am sure that over 60% of the population has some type of blood sugar disorder. A number of years ago I recall that I volunteered to speak on the subject of nutrition to Alcoholics Anonymous participants in a northeastern city. I remember being extremely annoyed, not because of any lack of interest, but because deserts and sugar filled coffee were being served during the recess. One day a retired Harvard professor took me aside and asked if I understood why these harmful substances were being served. I admitted I did not, so he then told me that it was well understood that all addicts were addicted primarily to sugar.

Shortly thereafter, I conducted research on the chemical composition of alcohol and found that the body identifies and utilizes all forms of alcohol as pure sugar. I do not mean to dismiss the eventual emotional connection that alcohol establishes with addiction, but, let me strongly state, an alcoholics' initial problem is sugar. This is why we see so many addicted fathers and mothers produce children who are predisposed to alcoholism.

Candida Albicans

Years ago I started to recognize that many of the guests at the Institute found their health improving greatly, while others had symptoms that seemed to block complete recovery. After many years of pondering this, we were never able to come up with a definitive reason. Then one day I came across a medical journal that mentioned candidiasis—and the answer to my search was suddenly revealed to me. The problem was called Candida Albicans.

Normal bacterial yeast that is found naturally everywhere in our external environment, is the culprit. We now know that because of a weakened immune system and an increased vulnerability to disease, these generally harmless fungi may invade one's body when this happens, our cells become de-oxygenated. In chronic cases, the yeast invades the organ tissues, such as the lungs and liver and generally creates an enormous health problem. It is an opportunistic lifeform that invades the weakened person. So often, when we are faced with cancer, diabetes, cardio-vascular illness and other such problems, Candida Albicans is also present and making it much more difficult for the individual to become healthy again.

Anyone who has been faced with this problem has probably heard hundreds of different opinions on what this disorder is, and how to deal with it. It is becoming a very popular disease and many pop-health authorities with little or no real experience with the problem are giving bad advice on the matter. Some of the worst advice regarding treatment through diet is that the sufferer should avoid anything with life in it and increase intake of animal foods. Through our practice, research and findings with this disease, the opposite is what is needed. Imagine the internal body when infected with Candida as a dank, moldy dripping cave and you would be imagining a rather accurate picture. When one has an enzyme deficient diet, and one's tissues are oxygen-starved through lack of exercise, one has unwittingly created an ideal environment for these fungi to multiply. The most effective way to clean up and rejuvenate the affected internal areas is to expose one's body to sunlight and air. Through eating a diet of raw unprocessed vegetables, germinated seeds, grains, nuts and beans, along with a regular exercise program, especially out of doors, this problem will certainly be overcome.

Common drugs used as a remedy for Candida Albicans are Nystatin and Nizoral (Ketoconazole) which, in both cases, weakens the immune system, the body's defense against invasive viruses, bacteria, yeasts, cancers, etc. The most difficult part of describing our truly effective treatment to a sufferer is when I have to tell the person that even in the best case scenario, it will take approximately a year and a half to regulate their system on a very orthodox Hippocrates program. There is no doubt that a larger percentage of the guests who attend the Institute are infected with this concern, and we must tailor their program accordingly.

Candida is closely related to hypoglycemia and diabetes, and this yeast infestation actually draws the blood sugar to feed itself. When you are experiencing any symptoms of hypoglycemia, recognize that your susceptibility to candida is greatly increased. Some of the symptoms of moderate candida are itchy nose and eyes, nasal drip, a congested throat, fatigue, anal itching, gas and bloating, foul oral or anal odor and a generally confused state of mind. Self-diagnosis is never 100% reliable so I suggest that you investigate this matter by locating an immunological blood testing facility that has a competent test procedure for candida.

If you wish to explore proven methods of eliminating this problem, you should attend our three week health program.

Chronic Fatigue/Fibromyalgia

These retro-virus menaces are thought to be mutations from other larger microbes which now have created a plague among the western population. In North America alone it is approximated that 40% of our youth below the age of 35 have some form of these potentially crippling new diseases. Everything from pain to disorientation on to sleeplessness and even the opposite, constant lethargy are some of the problems attributed to these newly evolved chronic diseases. First named Epstein/Barr it is now known that there is a wide variety of retroviruses that fit into this catch-basin called Chronic Fatigue/Fibromyalgia. We would venture to say that there are probably millions of newly formed microbes that your body is constantly attempting to keep under control that fall into this category. Often mistaken as severe depression and/or mental illness, there are hundreds of thousands who have been incorrectly treated with psychiatric medicines.

Observing the most dramatic cases, often bedridden, recovering, gives us complete confidence that a focused and dedicated individual who is willing to employ all necessary parts of a healthy life should never fret about Chronic Fatigue, Fibromyalgia or retro-viruses.

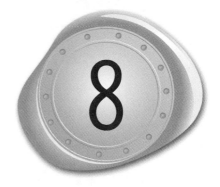

What to Expect
from Others

If you have serious health problems for which you have consulted a medical doctor you were probably told that a dietary program such as ours in ineffective. Society has been brainwashed by special interest groups (the food companies, the pharmaceutical companies and the medical associations) into an unquestioned acceptance of medical means as the only possible therapy that will work. These allopathically-trained M.D.'s are taught only to administer drugs, and surgeons will most often suggest surgery.

We embrace an eclectic approach to health and we utilize many tested and useful methods. For the most part, we suggest you avoid the use of unnecessary drugs. We feel that nutritious food is the best medicine, along with the sensible employment of supplements. We have found that the synergistic effect of prescription drugs is the most dangerous problem our guests have had to deal with. Some combinations of prescribed drugs can have lethal consequences. However, with certain illnesses, parasitic infections, for example, our physicians employ allopathic medicines.

At times we meet people who are quite skeptical, critical and sometimes even hostile regarding our program. We have found it is never wise to try to convince people who are openly antagonistic to our dietary approach to healing. Most people are not ready to give up their ethnic foods, their addictions and lifestyle or their monofocused faith in the medical faculty. The individual who lives this diet and expresses boundless health provides the most stunning proof that this lifestyle is effective.

In terms of what to expect during your detoxification period, we can offer a few guidelines. Actually, 60% of accumulated wastes will be released in the first seven days of your program, but complete healing and restoration of the body takes a number of years and breaks down into stages of 7 year increments. It will take the first seven years to completely rebuild the body in the following phases:

1 day–1½ years.......................... Digestive cleansing—major fat deposits and calcifications removed.

1½–2 years............................... Deep tissue cleansing & joint cleansing.

2–5 years.................................. Bone structure, cartilage and further joint cleansing.

5½–6 ¼ years........................... Organ repositioning and renewal.

6–7 years.................................. Brain tissue and neurological cleansing.

Cleansing reactions may ensue as layer after layer is stripped away. But you will feel better and better as time passes. Due to the body's cellular intelligence, every part is affected by the whole. When one part is renewed, this leads to greater integrity and harmony within the whole being.

During the second 7-year cycle, the emotional body is dealt with and refined. The third 7-year cycle brings out enhanced universal understanding, and a further understanding of your role in life.

• • •

**Become You and
everything will
normalize**

• • •

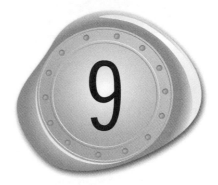

Individualizing
The Diet

One of the mistakes that any teacher or group leader makes in dispensing information and advice is becoming overzealous in treatment and making blanket statement that convey the impression that there is only one correct way to proceed.

At Hippocrates, we fell into these very traps and unconsciously exaggerated the effectiveness or appropriateness of a general program that was not individualized in any way. For decades now we have implemented a more open approach in dealing with any given situation. One of the gifts of nature is the uniqueness of each individual, and this holds true with our personal needs in renewing health. We should not disregard or discount valid information because our own concepts and experiences may differ. Choices may be the proper remedy, but dogmatism usually results in obstruction.

We have modified our stance to the point where we realize that the less desirable drug, operation or radiation therapy may be necessary in some cases. This is a decision that requires the most careful consideration.

Many people reading this book or who enroll in our Life Transformation Program follow a typical meat, dairy, poultry and fish diet, which also includes many processed foods. Although we may agree that such a diet is not health-giving, we are aware of the psychological attachments to former eating habits. In most cases where people are not in life-threatening situations, they can make a steady, unhurried change to a more healthful diet. An optimum diet may not be identical for everyone, but it should be obvious that all animal foods, processed sugars, flour, fats, commercial oil and excess proteins be eliminated. A good way to proceed is to map out a 6 month plan to reach your goal. Your first steps must be to eliminate your addictions to coffee, sugar, smoking, alcohol and drugs. The one "bad" thing you hold onto is always the biggest detriment to your health. Your wise choices will propel you into a heightened level of wellness.

The "quick fix" is an anomaly. It never fixes anything. Relying on a pill to take away the pain has been the western approach to self-medication. Common sense dictates that we discover the cause of our problems and eliminate them safely and effectively. The usual first step is to detoxify the body with a cleansing, nutritious diet. It is certainly not a rapid process. It is more like the seasons as they change—a gradual, definitive, long-lasting approach which will undeniably change your life and the way you deal with others. You can expect to emerge as a gentler, kinder, more compassionate individual as your emotional health is restored concurrently with your physical health.

Your oral fixations, deeply entrenched emotional traits and diminished spirit are all poor companions at the beginning of your road to recovery. You can be sure that your recovery has begun when your new companions are healthful eating habits, heightened self-esteem, happiness and an enlightened spirit.

Your obligation to yourself is to establish a goal, to proceed to that goal with determination, to embrace the goal and upon reaching it, to establish a new and higher goal. This applies to all areas of life, not only to your change of diet. Progress is a basic principle that governs life itself.

Longtime members of our organization are aware that the Hippocrates Health Institute has never advocated or recommended the use of supplements or vitamins as a dietary complement because we feel that a variety of whole, unprocessed and unheated foods are intrinsically superior, have a more balanced composition and can be more fully absorbed. However, after long experience, research and application, we now recommend certain supplements which are Living Food based. This expands and expedites the building and healing process.

Our research experiments on the utilization of enzymes in the last thirty years have shown us that they can provide an enormous boost in improved digestion and healing. We unequivocally recommend certain whole food algae, both the green single-celled and the blue-green varieties. The incredible nutrients and minerals they provide cannot be duplicated at this time in any land-based plants. Algae strengthen your RNA and DNA.

When people graduate from the Hippocrates program, for the rest of their lives, as a courtesy to them, we have our medical staff analyze their blood profiles and medical reports, so that we can continually refine and "tune up" their healing lifestyle. What one needs now maybe quite different in one, five or ten years from now. Health care must take a new approach creating life-long relationships with individuals. This, candidly, is the only way possible to effectively assist a person in their pursuit of a health filled life.

Since the inception of this approach, over the last three decades, we have been extremely pleased and fulfilled by the response from our alumnus in this newly-formed team approach to health. Given the ability to follow through not only makes the validity of the Living Foods program stronger, it also clearly places the responsibility on you to achieve your goal. As many of you have heard the stories about the Chinese physicians in the outreaches of the country who are only paid when people in the community are well, and not paid when they become sick, our western approach of making you act on your lifestyle achieves a similar goal. By taking back the power to heal yourself you are utilizing the most significant gift that human potential harbors.

• • •

**What one
needs now may be quite
different in one,
five or ten years**

• • •

• • •

**Your obligation to yourself
is to establish
a goal, to proceed
to that goal
with determination,
and upon reaching it,
establish a new
and higher goal**

• • •

Conclusion

This book represents a crystallized view of our multi-faceted focus. We have embraced life fully and, as a result, we are enjoying life and health enthusiastically. Our methods are not complex – they are the dynamics of living itself.

Rather than leave you with a redundant summation, we prefer to list some thought provoking statements that will hopefully lead you into the path of true health.

Food

Coffee drinking is not an innocuous habit but a harmful addiction.

Alcohol is one of the most harmful products that is unrestricted by governments.

A sunflower green is complete, perfect protein food.

Eating starches and proteins together creates a sulfur compound in the body causing gas.

Peanut butter has been shown to be carcinogenic due to the mold, aflatoxin, often found on the nuts.

If you must use a sugary substance, "Stevia" is the most natural and not harmful. Remember, sugar of any kind feeds illness.

• •

Caffeine, as in soda, coffee, etc., is a dangerous drug just like cocaine, heroin and morphine and is responsible for weakening the nervous system causing cardiac irregularities and increasing the risk of pancreatic cancer.

• •

Ripe strawberry juice has been found to eliminate fatty deposits from muscles and to restore elasticity to the skin.

• •

Chick peas, first sprouted and then cooked, are nutritious and non-gas forming. They are a good choice in any transition diet.

• •

Phytonutrients are the most important nutritional discovery in history.

• •

Vegetables from the "nightshade" family such as peppers, tomatoes, potatoes or eggplant, should not be cooked and should be consumed ripe.

• •

Boron, found most extensively in legumes, fruits and vegetables, may be a key factor in preventing osteoporosis.

• •

Billions of years ago the blue-green algae produced the oxygen in our atmosphere. These algae, with their countless years of cell memory, help our cells to remember their perfect functioning.

• •

Fermented drinks, once a part of the Hippocrates diet, have been eliminated due to research showing that it encouraged the growth of unfriendly bacteria, which negated the effects of good bacteria. Mounting complaints of discomfort prompted us to delete these fermented drinks from our diet. Saurkraut juice is a stable and health producing beverage.

• •

Body

In a toxic body, poisonous acids build up in the blood, leading to joint erosion and cause a host of certain diseases.

Eat only when your appetite tells you to do so. Eating when angry, anxious or fearful contributes to constipation & mal-absorption.

The human body must have daily stimulation through exercise, fresh air and sunshine to function in a normal manner.

The human body completely regenerates within a seven-year period.

Lifestyle play more of a role today than ever before in human illness, due to massive destruction to which we have exposed our systems in the last decades.

Bathing should be done a minimum of every 24 hours. If one really wishes to clean one's body, taking saunas, steam baths, or using a whirlpool are excellent choices to further cleansing.

Eating a completely raw, live food diet results in weight reduction, and research has shown that a well-nourished body functions much more efficiently and has a greater resiliency to environmental and emotional dangers.

When maintaining a live food diet, one must engage in muscular resistance exercises to develop muscular strength, improve cardiovascular action and stamina. Muscle is the only weight we want on our body.

Mental & Spiritual

Never stop learning. Keep your mind elastic and teachable. Don't be a "know-it-all".

Prepare your food with gratitude and appreciation.

When the ego is in charge, it is like the tail wagging the dog.

When the vision is in your heart, you are home free.

Spirituality is not a set of rules and regulations that constrict or limit us. It is really the totality of endless potential.

Success is established, built, created and maintained through consistency, commitment, focus, faith and knowledge.

There is overwhelming proof that the mind affects every part of the human anatomy.

Sexism, racism and prejudices are due to our lack of knowledge, information and self-esteem.

Environment

Wear only natural fabrics like organic cotton, linen, hemp and silk if possible. Man-made fabrics can give off fumes.

The present wool sheering process is often cruel and exploitative, so use your judgment when choosing woolen clothing.

92% of the world is under nourished, but a plant-based world would assure everybody adequate food and nourishment.

• •

The toxic fumes which escape when you fill your gas tank are absorbed by your clothing and are later released into the air in your home. Some gas stations have signs suggesting that you not stand close and that you turn your face away as you fill your tank.
• •

Eating some "fast foods" can mean destroying part of the earth's rainforests.
• •

Asbestos, radon gas, high tension wires, fumes radiating from plastics and man-made materials, electronic waves, etc. have all added to the constant bombardment of our immune and cellular systems.
• •

Noise levels distract even the most centered person, so we should provide ourselves with daily rest periods of quiet relaxation.
• •

Stress is always thought of as external forces affecting you. An improved self-image will create the self-confidence needed to deal effectively with any stressful situation.
• •

The American Cancer Society has announced that they foresee an annual death rate of many more than one million people if the problems of environmental pollution and chemically contaminated foods are not remedied and eliminated.
• •

Sleep only on 100% cotton or organic cotton sheets. Luxurious pure silk sheets are also healthful. Your skin absorbs and is affected by everything it touches, and the chemicals in polyester fabrics are toxic. They also emit fumes which are harmful to our respiratory system.
• •

The same water that is here today is the original that was here at the beginning of the earth.
• •

Compost when possible to build soil and enrich the Planet.
• •

Recycle everything to reduce waste, energy usage and pollution.
• •

••

MTBE, a gasoline additive, which has now seeped into the water systems in many parts of the world, has been found to be the most cancer causing chemical ever researched. Distilled or distilled and molecularly organized water are the only choices which rid us of this mutagen.

••

Walk, bicycle or use electric, hybrid, or hydrogen vehicles to reach your destination.

••

Planting native foliage and trees around your homes and businesses will decrease water usage and increase air pollution reducing oxygen.

••

Reduce your cell phone and computer usage to the minimum thus avoiding unnecessary energy output and potential disease causing emissions.

••

When possible, take a day of rest from all appliances, television, electronics, recorded music and transportation giving yourself the time and opportunity to take a walk with friends or family, collecting discarded debris in your neighborhoods, parks, beaches and cities.

••

Purchase wind generated electric technology for your homes and business use whenever possible. This cutting edge equipment will become increasingly available as time passes, dramatically reducing environmental pollution and economic output.

••

Hippocrates Offers An Unsurpassed Health Program

At the start of the 21st Century Hippocrates was internationally distinguished as North America's foremost Complimentary Health Center. Lifestyle changes permanently applied by thousands to help them battle disease, extend their lives and establish the highest level of energy possible, are just a few reasons people attend. Whatever your reason, we invite you to come to our in-house guest program which will teach you how to implement this lifestyle into your daily routine. For several decades people have been acquiring the needed education and motivation to change their inappropriate habits through spending this valuable time with us. Twenty-one days is the usual length of our program but longer or shorter stays can be arranged. For information please call or write to our program counselors at:

Hippocrates Health Institute
1466 Hippocrates Way
West Palm Beach, FL 33411
Tel: (561)471-8876
Fax: (561)471-2979
www.hippocratesinst.com
info@hippocratesinst.com

Hippocrates Therapy Building
Offerings and Open House

The Hippocrates Life Transformation Program is intimate and requires the environmental sanctuary of our facility and grounds to nurture our participants. There are two ways that the general public can learn more and participate in limited activities on the Hippocrates campus.

First, two times a week there are tours offered, times and scheduling may change so by calling 561-471-8876, you will be informed as to when you can share in this activity. In the last week of each month there is an "Open House" held which includes a tour, lecture and question and answer session and food sampling. Call 561-471-8876 for reservations.

Hippocrates Oasis Spa offers a wide array of professional services from the most highly skilled therapists with an average of twenty years of acclaimed work in their fields. At times there is limited space for those people who are not participating in the program to come and share a little bit of what is part of the program. Please call the Oasis Spa at 561-471-5867 to explore the possibilities of your involvement at Hippocrates Health Institute.

Health Educator Certification

S tudents of all ages and from all corners of the globe awaken and develop their sense of passion and purpose while participating in our Hippocrates Health Educator Program. With roots dating back more than 30 years, the program prepares students to carry on Drs. Brian and Anna Maria Clement's work of educating people in a living foods lifestyle and the importance of naturopathic self-healing. Students are taught how to take a mind-body-spirit approach to foster positive lifestyle changes in themselves and others. The internationally acclaimed 9 week program provides the tools and connection necessary to become an active agent of change in the world of health. Upon graduation, our "Certified Hippocrates Health Educators" have written books, produced documentaries, organized retreats, created food or juice products, grown sprouts and wheatgrass for the community, become speakers or advocates of health or opened cafes. Others are working with people in their homes, creating public awareness through event planning or referring groups of people to Hippocrates in order to bring about health and happiness. The value of this program comes not only in the exposure to the how and why, but in the experience and synergy that is created when you surround yourself with like-minded people from around the world, 50 acres of natural beauty and the entirety of the living food lifestyle as taught at Hippocrates. It is offered three times a year, in the spring, summer and fall and if you are interested in applying or learning more details you can call (561)471-8876 x2110 or email healthed@hippocratesinst.org.

63

Life Transformation Program

Guests from all over the world benefit from health and nutritional counseling, non-invasive remedial and youth-enhancing therapies, state of the art spa services, inspiring talks on life principles and a tantalizing daily buffet of enzyme-rich, organic meals. Health-minded people attend the program in equal numbers to those who visit to reverse disease. For those who are new to the living food lifestyle, the Hippocrates Life Transformation Program makes this a comfortable transition. The medical team and professional care servers support guests as they transform their lives in an encouraging environment, along with others who are recovering from similar challenges. HHI alumni are people from all walks of life who have benefited from the institute's blueprint. They share stories of recovery that are considered miraculous by some, but are actually quite typical of people who have embraced the Hippocrates lifestyle. After graduating, alumni are afforded the privilege of periodic, lifelong, written counsel. For over half a century, Hippocrates Health Institute has helped people prevent and reverse disease as well as the premature aging process.

Equipment Needed to Implement The Live Food Program

There are a number of items which are essential for anyone wishing to incorporate the live food program into their daily routine. The items listed below can be found at the Hippocrates Store, or ordered through Mail Order or on our Web store.

Sprouting Supplies
- Trays with and without holes
- Hydrosol rack to hold trays
- Easy sprouter and sprouting lids
- Sprouting mats and sprouting bags
- Seeds
- Plant remineralizer

Kitchen Equipment and Supplies
- Single Auger electric juicer (manual juicer is optional)
- Food dehydrator and paraflex dehydrator sheets

- Blender for making nut milks and dressings
- Mandolin slicers
- Spiral slicers
- Green bags

Water Systems
- Reverse Osmosis Living Water System
- Steam distilled water system
- Shower filter systems

Personal Health Care
- Enema bags, catheter and bulb syrings
- Dry brush
- Oral irrigator and tongue scraper
- All natural personal care products

All items available online at hippocratesinst.com or call 561-471-8876

Hippocrates
Publications

Books by *Dr. Anna Maria Clement*

#1   A Families' Guide to Health & Healing

#2   Healthful Cuisine

#3   The Power of a Woman with *Katherine Powell*

Books by *Dr. Brian Clement*

#1   7 Keys to Lifelong Sexual Vitality
      With *Dr. Anna Maria Clement*

#2   Dairy Deception

#3   Food is Medicine, Volumes I, II, III

#4   Killer Clothes

#5   Killer Fish

#6   LifeForce; Superior Health and Longevity

#7   Living Foods for Optimum Health

#8   Longevity: Enjoying Long Life

#9   Supplements Exposed

Hippocrates Publications Series for Living

#1   Hippocrates Health Program
      By *Brian R. Clement*

#2   Belief, Integrity in Relationships
      By *Brian R. Clement & Katherine Powell*

#3   Children, the Ultimate Creation
      By *Drs. Anna Maria & Brian R. Clement*

#4   Exercise: Creating Your Persona
      By *Brian R. Clement*

#5   Relationships: Voyages Through Life
      By *Drs. Anna Maria & Brian R. Clement*

#6   Spirituality in Healing and Life
      By *Brian R. Clement*

HIPPOCRATES HEALTH INSTITUTE
1466 Hippocrates Way
West Palm Beach, FL 33411
TEL: 561)471-8876
FAX: (561)471-9646
www.hippocratesinst.com
info@hippocratesinst.com

Footnotes

Introduction

1. Robbins, John. Diet for a New America
   Walpole NH Still point Publishing 1987

Chapter 1

1. Kulvinskas, Viktoras. Survival Into the 21st Century
   Woodstock Valley CT/Fairfield, IA
   21st Century Publications 1975

2. Cousens, Gabriel. Spiritual Nutrition and the Rainbow Diet
   Boulder CO
   Cassandra Press, 1986

3. Kouchakoff, Paul. The Influence of Cooking
   On the Blood Formula of Man
   Proceedings, First International Congress
   Of Micro-biology, Paris, 1930

4. Howell, Edward. Food Enzymes for Health and Longevity
   Woodstock Valley, CT
   Omangod Press, 1946

Chapter 2

1. Wigmore, Ann, Hippocrates Live Food Program
   Boston, MA Hippocrates Press, 1984

Chapter 4

1. Kime, Zane R. Sunlight, Panryn, CA
   World Health Publications, 1980

2. VDT News, Vol. III, No.4 July/Aug.,1986
   PO Box 1799, Grand Central Station
   New York, NY 10162

ALL OF THE BOOKS
REFERENCED IN THESE
FOOTNOTES ARE
RECOMMENDED
READING

● ● ●

A health filled life
will create
the foundation which
brings you
the ability to
embrace complete happiness

● ● ●